THERE IS

NO LIGHT

WITHOUT

DARKNESS

The
NOCTURNAL
JOURNAL

A LATE-NIGHT EXPLORATION OF WHAT'S REALLY ON YOUR MIND

LEE CRUTCHLEY

A TARCHERPERIGEE BOOK

tarcherperigee

An imprint of Penguin Random House LLC
375 Hudson Street
New York, New York 10014

TarcherPerigee with tp colophon is a registered trademark of
Penguin Random House LLC.

Most TarcherPerigee books are available at special quantity discounts for
bulk purchase for sales promotions, premiums, fund-raising, and educational
needs. Special books or book excerpts also can be created to fit specific
needs. For details, write: SpecialMarkets@penguinrandomhouse.com.

ISBN 9780143130796

Printed in the United States of America
1 3 5 7 9 10 8 6 4 2

Book design by Lee Crutchley

FOR ALL THE DREAMERS
(AND ALL THE DREAMS)

THERE

DARK

WITHOU

IS NO

NESS

T LIGHT

nocturnal
/näkˈtərnl/

ADJECTIVE

DONE, OCCURRING, OR ACTIVE AT NIGHT.
"MOST OWLS ARE NOCTURNAL."

INTRODUCTION

I should start by saying that this book won't help you to sleep any better, or even at all. But it will help you to make better use of those hours when you can't sleep. The hours when you're so full of angst and worries that you can't really switch off at night (like me), or haunted by dark thoughts that you don't always understand (like me), or repeatedly woken up right at the point of nodding off by yet another amazing idea (like me).

No matter what is causing your lack of sleep, it almost always stems from the same reason. In the modern world it's hard to find, make, or allow enough time to really connect with yourself. The days are becoming busier and busier, and this means that your worries get suppressed, your feelings stay unexplored, and your most creative ideas remain itches that you don't have the time to scratch. All of this floods your brain the moment you try to switch off for the night, and there is a good reason for that.

The night is the perfect time to explore those thoughts, feelings, and ideas. Under the cover of darkness you're free to think thoughts you dare not think, feel emotions you're afraid to feel, and talk to yourself without feeling crazy. While this book won't help you to sleep any better, it will hopefully help you to live a little better. It will provide you with a place to shelter from the gaze and opinions of others and allow you to reconnect with the most important, but often most neglected, person in your life—you.

There are so many things that can keep you from sleeping, it's a wonder you ever actually get to sleep at all. It can be easy to let one (or all) of these things become obstructions that rule your night and block you from sleep. But if you decide to accept and explore those late-night thoughts and feelings, rather than succumb to them, you're often able to see them from a fresh perspective. Hidden doors are revealed in obstructions that once felt like walls, as the darkness illuminates them, and you, in a way that the light cannot.

OBSTRUCTION

WHERE ARE YOU ON THESE SCALES?

RIGID   ADAPTABLE

SELFISH   SELFLESS

INDIFFERENT   IN LOVE

INTROVERT   EXTROVERT

RELAXED   WIRED

USE A DIFFERENT COLOR OR SHAPE
TO INDICATE WHERE YOU'D LIKE TO BE

REALITY IMAGINATION

REACTIVE PROACTIVE

PESSIMIST OPTIMIST

SAFE SCARED

THE PAST THE FUTURE

TURN OUT THE LIGHTS AND DRAW
WHAT KEEPS YOU AWAKE AT NIGHT

IT'S LATE AND YOUR PHONE IS BUZZING. WHO IS IT AND WHAT DO THEY WANT?

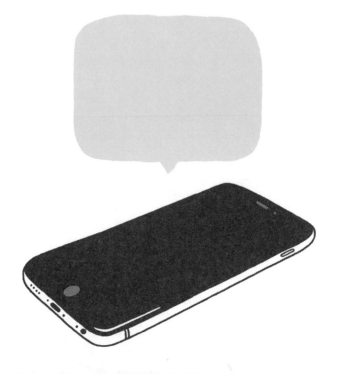

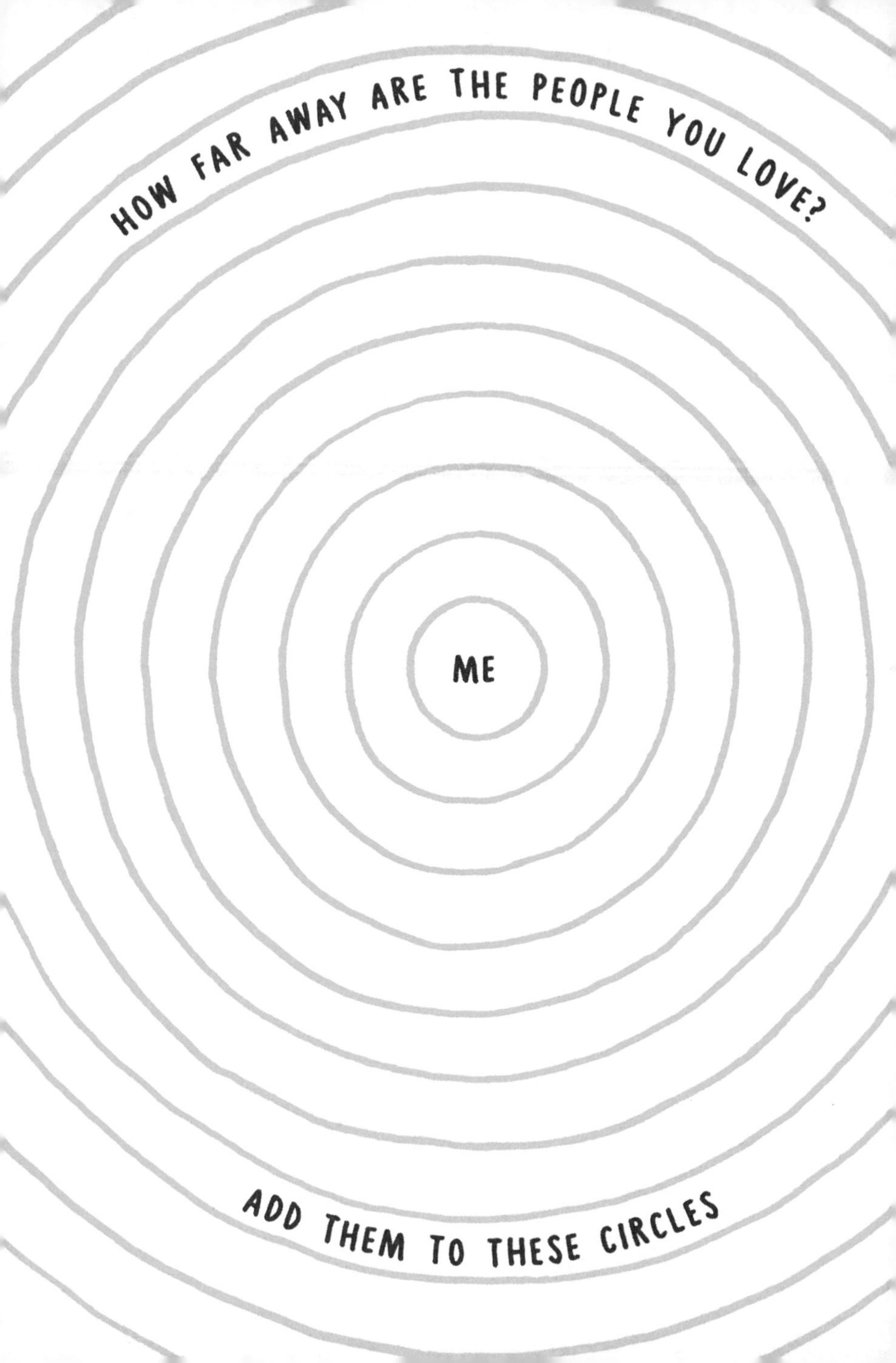

HOW FAR AWAY ARE THE PEOPLE YOU LOVE?

ME

ADD THEM TO THESE CIRCLES

IMPORTANT THOUGHTS

UNIMPORTANT THOUGHTS

WHAT'S THE SINGLE
MOST IMPORTANT THING
ON YOUR MIND RIGHT NOW?

WRITE IT DOWN AND KEEP IT IN A PLACE THAT YOU'LL SEE IT OFTEN:

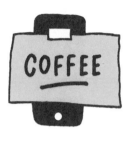

STUCK TO YOUR PHONE

IN YOUR PURSE

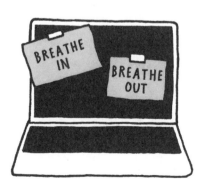

OR ON YOUR COMPUTER

WHAT GETS YOU OUT OF BED EACH MORNING?

WHAT SENDS YOU TO SLEEP?

THINK OF THE BIGGEST QUESTION ON YOUR MIND

CLOSE YOUR EYES

POINT TO AN ANSWER

HA HA HA
HA HA
HA

I DOUBT
II

100%
YES

OF COURSE!
JK

IT'S
50-50

I
HOPE SO

404

UMM...

YOU
KNOW
BETTER

IT'S IN YOUR
HANDS

NOPE, SORRY

WHEN YOU ARE READY

IT'S A NO, OR YES, OR MAYBE

IT'S CERTAIN (PROBABLY)

INTENTIONALLY BLANK

GOOGLE KNOWS ALL

THE ANSWER IS ICE CREAM

42

ASK AGAIN TOMORROW

YES (HONESTLY)

I CAN'T SEE WHY NOT

IS THAT A TRICK QUESTION?

REPEAT THIS WHENEVER YOU NEED TO

WRITE A RÉSUMÉ THAT CONSISTS
ONLY OF YOUR FAILURES AND REJECTIONS

DATE	EVENT

WHICH OF THESE ARE STILL HOLDING YOU BACK?

THE PAST...

THE PRESENT...

THE FUTURE...

WHAT ARE THE THREE HEAVIEST THINGS IN YOUR LIFE, AND WHAT GIVES THEM SO MUCH WEIGHT?

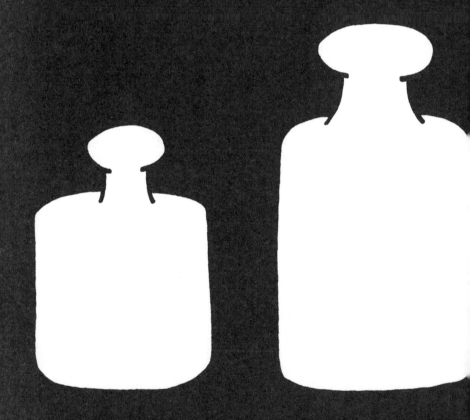

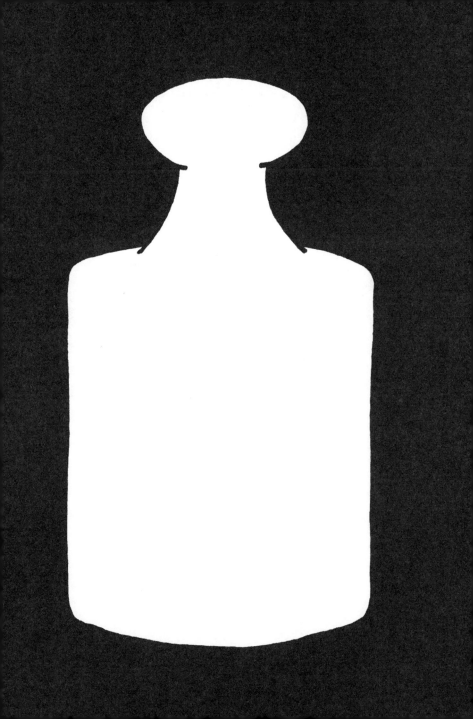

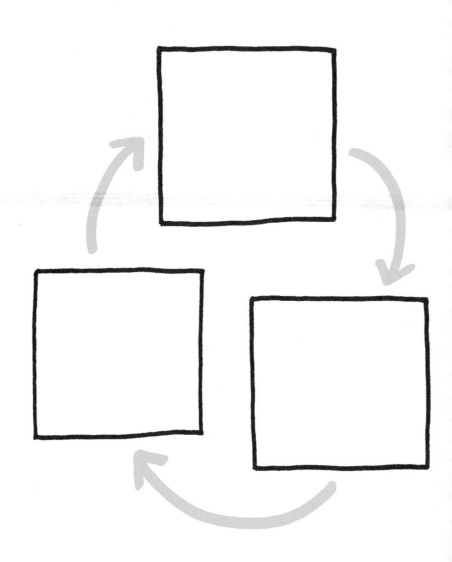

WHAT CYCLE ARE YOU CAUGHT IN?

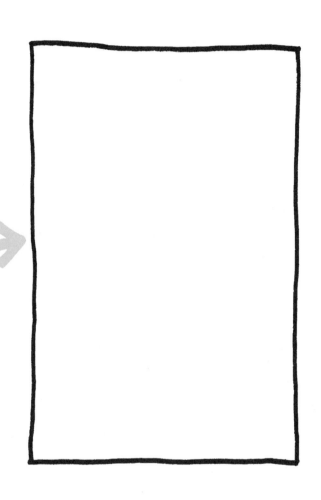

WHAT CAN YOU DO TO BREAK OUT OF IT?

WRITE A LETTER OF FORGIVENESS

THE LAST TIME I...

CRIED:

LIED:

LAUGHED SO HARD IT HURT:

ID SOMETHING IMPORTANT:

AID THANK YOU:

AID I LOVE YOU:

WHAT MAKES YOU FEEL...

AFRAID

RRAVF

ASHAMED

PROUD

ALONE

UNDERSTOOD

APATHY

EMPATHY

SADNESS

HAPPINESS

HATE

LOVE

WHAT DO YOU WANT?

CROSS THAT OUT. OK, WHAT DO YOU WANT?

YOU'RE GETTING THERE, BUT CROSS THAT OUT TOO.

NE LAST TIME, WHAT DO YOU REALLY WANT?

KAY, IT'S GOOD TO BE SURE!

WHY YOU

ARE

HERE?

The thing about finding hidden doors is that it's generally terrifying to actually walk through them, because you never know what will be on the other side. But when you actually confront your fears they're rarely as scary as they first seem. Exploring your fears in more depth will often reveal things that you didn't even know you thought, felt, or wanted (as well as a few skeletons). There's a reason children ask the question "Why?" hundreds of times a day. It's how they learn, grow, and move forward. The darkness is the best time to ask yourself what you're really afraid of, and why.

FEAR

WHEN WAS THE LAST TIME YOU WERE AFRAID?

EMBARRASSING
TO ADMIT

NEAR-DEATH
EXPERIENCE

HOW SCARY WAS IT?

DO YOU BELIEVE IN GOD?

WHAT WAS THE BIGGEST DECISION YOU MADE TODAY?

LITERALLY
THE WORST

COULDN'T HAVE
GONE BETTER

HOW DID YOU DO?

DO YOU BELIEVE IN YOURSELF?

FILL THIS BOX WITH
ALL OF YOUR WORRIES

NOW SORT THEM INTO THESE BOXES

PRODUCTIVE WORRIES

UNPRODUCTIVE WORRIES

HOW WOULD YOU SPEND TOMORROW
IF THERE WERE NO TO-DO LIST?

HIGHLIGHT ANY THINGS YOU COULD
INTEGRATE INTO YOUR DAILY LIFE

WRITE A TO-DO LIST FOR TOMORROW THAT CONTAINS AT LEAST ONE OF THESE THINGS

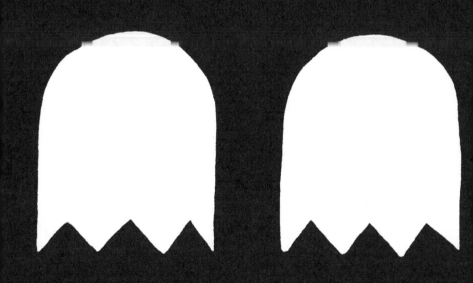

WHAT GHOSTS FROM THE PAST
ARE STILL HAUNTING YOU?

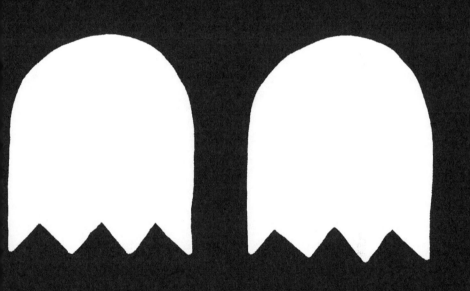

WHAT WOULD YOU DO IF FEAR DIDN'T EXIST?
AT WORK I WOULD:

IN LOVE I WOULD:

N THE FUTURE I WOULD:

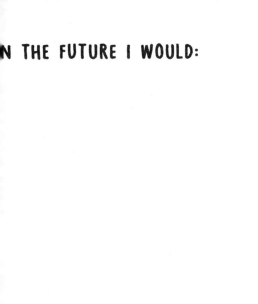

IGHT NOW I WOULD:

WHAT IS YOUR BIGGEST FEAR FOR THE FUTURE?

HOW LIKELY IS IT TO COME TRUE?

WHAT CAN YOU DO TO STOP IT?

IF YOU CAN'T STOP IT, HOW CAN YOU ACCEPT IT?

IN MOMENTS OF DARKNESS, WHAT DO YOU SEE?

USE A WHITE CRAYON OR PENCIL

THINGS TO AVOID FOREVER

THINGS TO OVERCOME

WHAT'S CAUSING THAT FEELING
DEEP IN YOUR STOMACH?

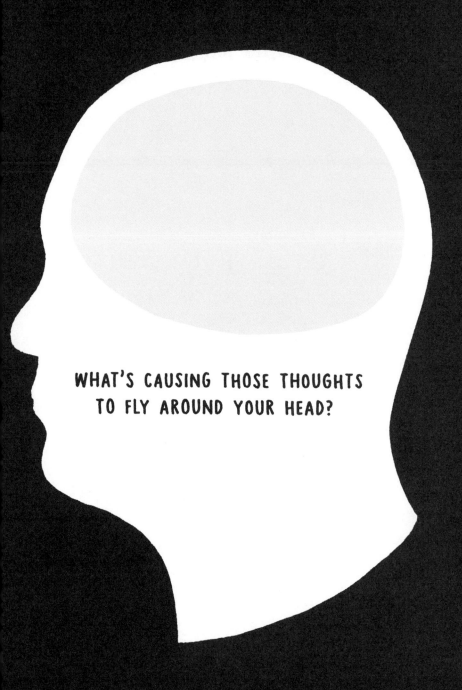

LIST EVERY TIME YOU FELT AFRAID, WORRIED, OR ANXIOUS TODAY

LIST EVERY TIME YOU FELT BRAVE, CONFIDENT, OR CALM TODAY

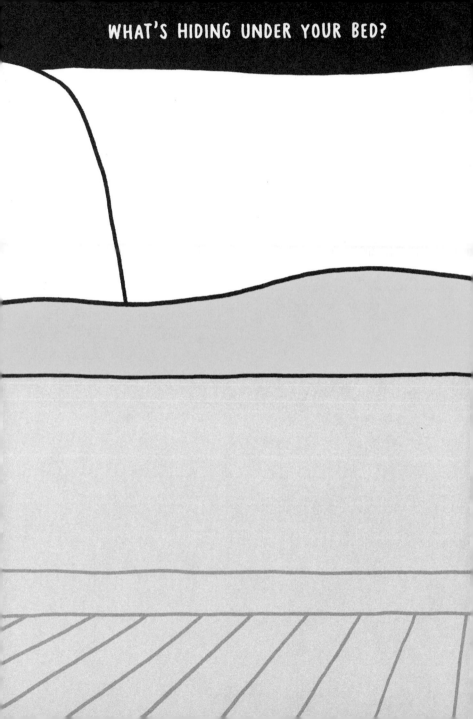

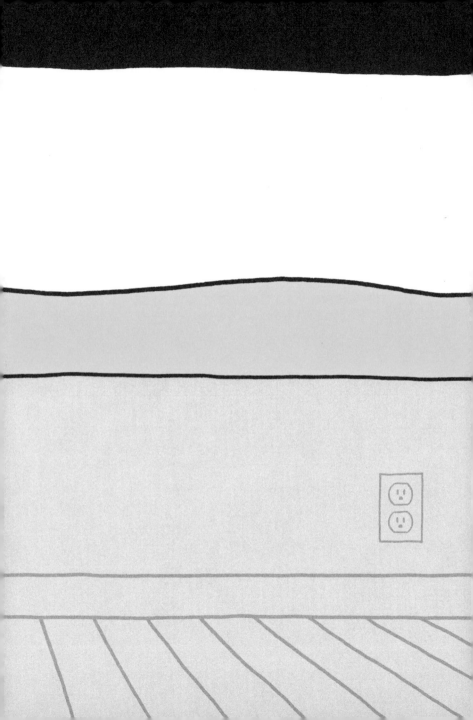

FILL THIS PAGE WITH DARK WORDS

DARK

FILL THIS PAGE WITH LIGHT WORDS

ONNECT THE TWO SIDES IN A WAY THAT FEELS RIGHT

WHAT'S THE SCARIEST THING YOU'VE EVER DONE?

WHAT'S THE SCARIEST THING YOU'LL EVER DO?

WHAT DO YOU THINK ARE THE TEN
MOST IMPORTANT QUESTIONS IN LIFE?

MARK THIS PAGE SOMEHOW. YOU'LL COME BACK TO THESE QUESTIONS LATER.

1:

2:

3:

4:

5:

6:

7:

8:

9:

10:

WHAT'S ONE THING YOU'D LOVE TO DO BUT ARE TOO SCARED TO TELL ANYONE ABOUT?

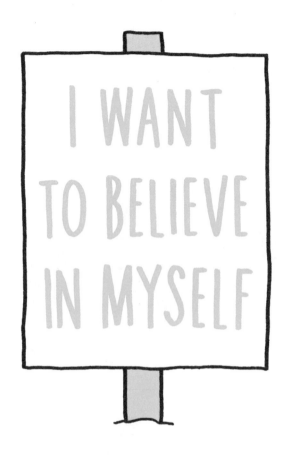

MAKE A SIGN TO ADVERTISE THIS SECRET
AMBITION AND DISPLAY IT ANONYMOUSLY
IN A PLACE WHERE OTHERS WILL SEE IT

WHAT A

AFRAI

RE YOU

D OF?

An often frustrating side effect of your brain winding down for the night is that you can become energized with inspiration and flooded with great ideas. This heightened creative state is not just a trick of the night. Your brain has relaxed its filters, you're becoming detached from your surroundings, and you're heading into the strange space that exists somewhere between being awake and being asleep. The ideas you have in this state can seem weird, and some may not even make sense in the morning, but magic can occur in those moments. When your mind gets off the beaten track and begins to wander along its own path, you should encourage it to keep going.

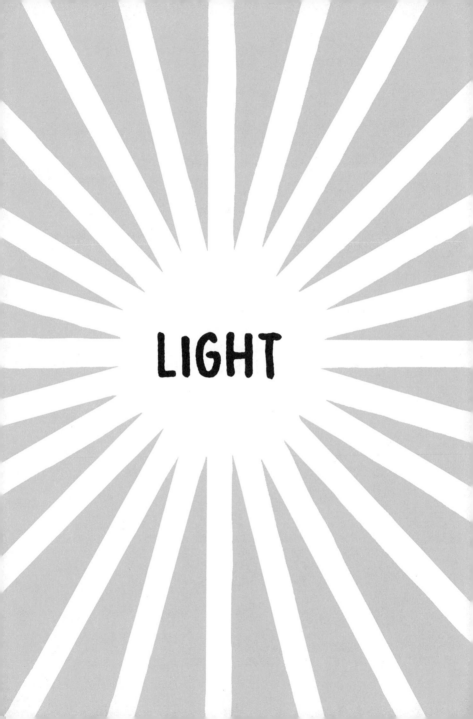

HOW AWAKE ARE YOU?

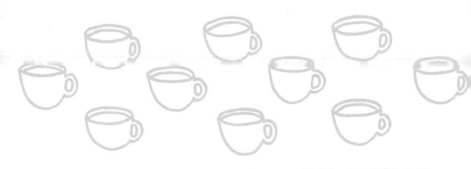

HOW MUCH CAFFEINE DID YOU HAVE TODAY?

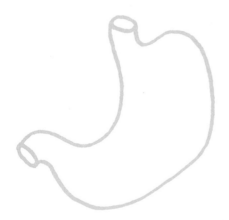 

HOW FULL IS
YOUR STOMACH?

HOW MANY HOURS
HAVE YOU SPENT
LOOKING AT SCREENS?

THREE WORDS TO DESCRIBE YOURSELF

WHAT'S ON
YOUR PIZZA?

WHAT DOES THE
FUTURE LOOK LIKE?

THREE WORDS TO DESCRIBE
THE PERSON YOU WANT TO BE

THINK OF SOMETHING COMPLETELY
UNRELATED TO EACH OF THESE WORDS

HORSE

TURQUOISE

CHURCH

FISH

MOUNTAIN

PIZZA

TWELVE

MIRROR

NEW YORK

PERSON

FILL THIS PAGE WITH MADE-UP WORDS

FLASHICOOL

PERTIFLEX

CHOOSE YOUR FAVORITES AND DEFINE THEM

MY DREAM...
PERSON:

PLACE:

HING:

IFE:

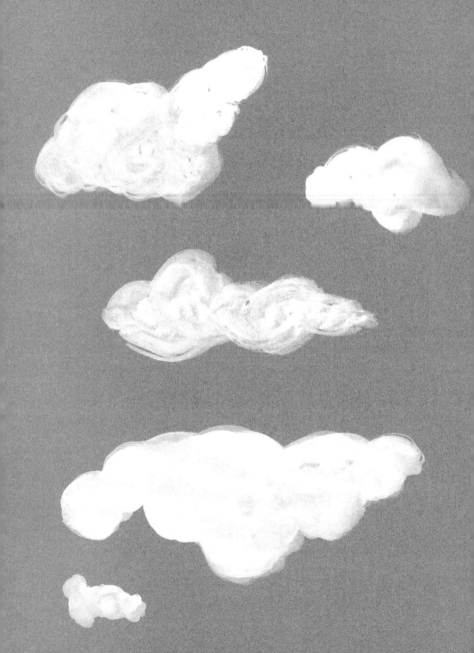

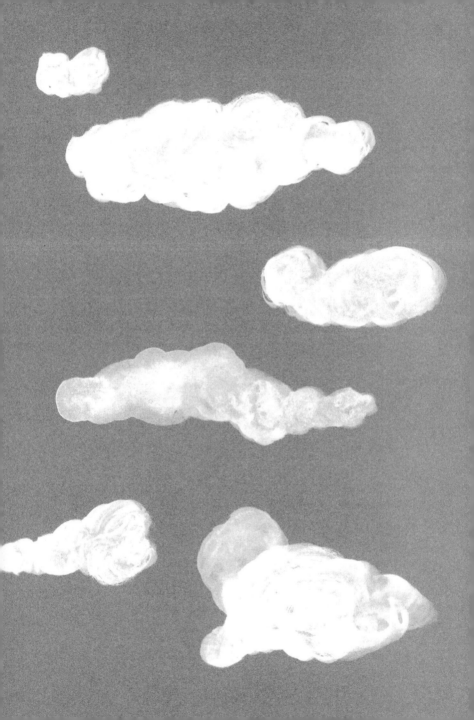

WHAT ARE YOUR THREE MAIN PROBLEMS RIGHT NOW?

1:

2:

3:

INVENT THINGS TO FIX EACH OF THEM
(DON'T WORRY ABOUT THE SCIENCE)

1:

2:

3:

NOW SEEMS LIKE A GOOD TIME
FOR SOME "ADULT COLORING"

THERE'S NOTHING FOR YOU TO COLOR; JUST START AND SEE WHAT HAPPENS

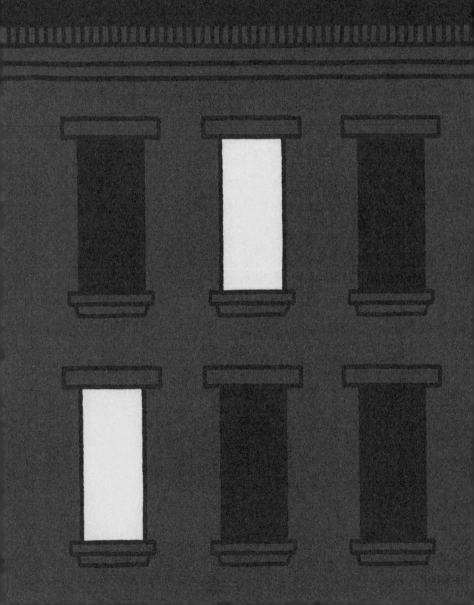

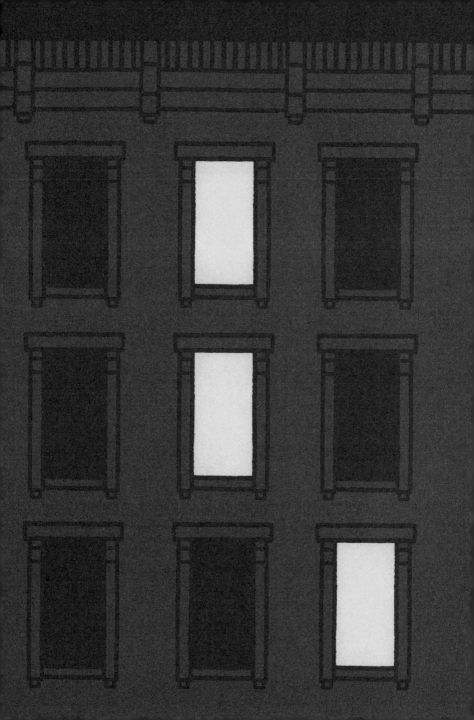

WRITE DOWN EVERY AMAZING IDEA **YOU** HAVE TONIGHT

OMORROW, HIGHLIGHT THE IDEAS THAT ARE STILL AMAZING

WRITE A LETTER ASKING YOUR CHILDHOOD HERO FOR ADVICE

WRITE ABOUT THE LAST TIME YOU...

TRIED A NEW FOOD

FOUND SOMETHING NEW IN YOUR TOWN

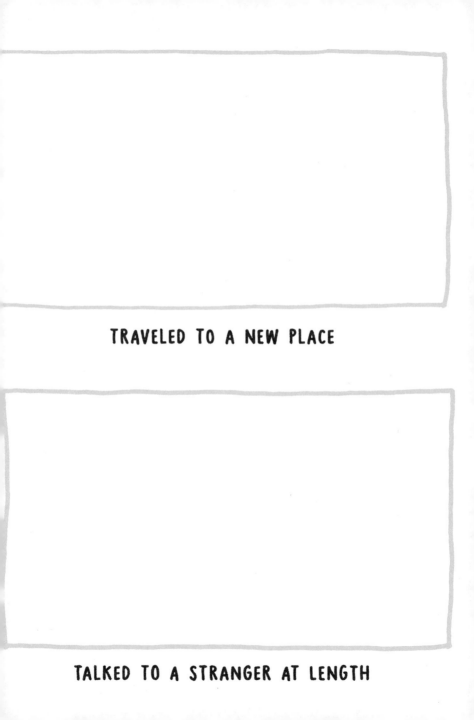

TRAVELED TO A NEW PLACE

TALKED TO A STRANGER AT LENGTH

FIND A RANDOM PHOTO AND STICK IT HERE

GOOD PLACES TO FIND RANDOM PHOTOS ARE:
THE FLOOR, THE INTERNET, OR PRINT ONE
OF MINE AT RANDOMPIC.LEECRUTCHLEY.COM

WHAT'S THE MOST AMAZING
THING YOU'VE EVER SEEN?

WHAT'S THE MOST AMAZING
THING YOU'VE NEVER SEEN?

CONNECT THE STARS TO MAKE YOUR OWN CONSTELLATIONS

WRITE ABOUT THREE GOOD THINGS

WHAT WILL BE YOUR GREATEST ACHIEVEMENT?

WHAT WILL BE YOUR FAVORITE PLACE?

WHO WILL YOU BE IN LOVE WITH?

WHAT WILL BE THE WORST THING YOU EVER DO?

WHAT WILL BE THE BEST THING YOU EVER DO?

WILL EVERYTHING BE OK IN THE END?

WHER
YOU G

E ARE

OING?

The darkness is a strange place where you can feel either absolutely terrified or completely safe, sometimes both at once. The darkness will often encourage you to feel your darkest feelings and think your darkest thoughts. Human instinct means you will usually be inclined to turn away from that darkness. But it's important to be brave and to confront it, maybe even prod and provoke it a little. By examining your shadow self in more depth you will realize that having dark thoughts does not (automatically) make you a dark person. There is no light without darkness.

THE WORST...
FOOD YOU'VE EATEN:

PERSON YOU'VE MET:

LIE YOU'VE TOLD:

WORDS YOU'VE SAID:

THOUGHT YOU'VE HAD:

THING YOU'VE DONE:

HOW DOES THE MOON FEEL TONIGHT?

HOW DO YOU FEEL TONIGHT?

PUT YOUR THUMB OVER THIS SEED
AND THINK OF EVERYTHING BAD.

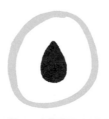

FEEL THE BAD THOUGHTS CIRCLE
AND BUILD UNTIL THEY FEEL SOLID.

NOW START TO PUSH THEM OUT OF YOUR MIND.

FEEL THEM FLOW DOWN THROUGH YOUR NECK,
INTO YOUR SHOULDER, ALONG YOUR ARM,
AND OUT THROUGH YOUR THUMB.

INTO THE SEED.

KEEP YOUR BAD THOUGHTS
FLOWING UNTIL YOU FEEL EMPTY.

DRAW YOUR ANSWERS TO THESE QUESTIONS

WHO DO YOU BLAME?

WHAT CAUSED THAT SCAR?

WHO DO YOU MISS?

WHAT HAPPENS WHEN WE DIE?

WHAT WOULD YOU
LIKE TO BURY FOREVER?

WRITE A LETTER TO SOMEONE YOU'VE LOST

~~RIHANNA~~

UGH

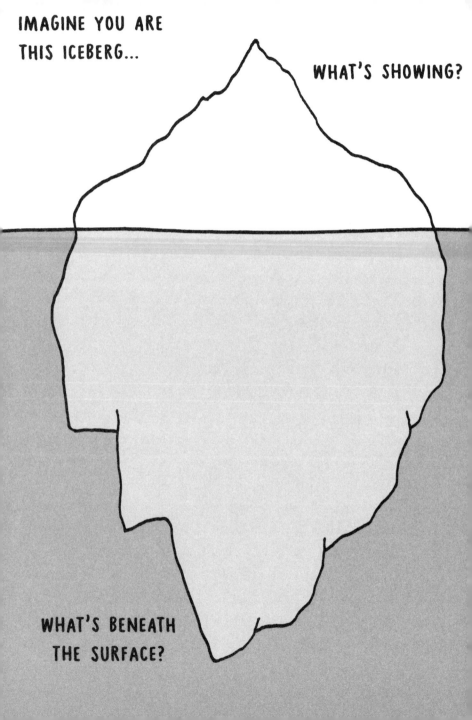

WHAT KEEPS YOU AFLOAT?

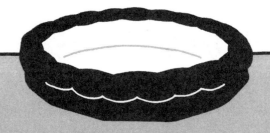

WHAT'S LURKING IN THE DEEP?

WRITE YOUR BLUEST THOUGHTS WITH YOUR BLUEST PEN

DESCRIBE YOUR FAVORITE PHYSICAL FEATURE

TURN OUT THE LIGHTS AND LOOK AT
THEM BOTH WITH A FLASHLIGHT

WHAT WERE YOUR THREE BIGGEST MISTAKES?

AND WHAT CAN YOU LEARN FROM THEM?

IF IT WERE POSSIBLE TO ERASE A SPECIFIC MEMORY, WOULD YOU DO IT?

YES   NO

IF YOU ANSWERED YES, GATHER THESE TWO THINGS AND MOVE ON TO THE NEXT PAGE

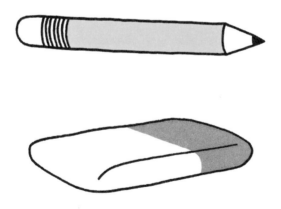

IF YOU ANSWERED NO, SERIOUSLY?

WRITE THE MEMORY IN AS MUCH DETAIL
AS YOU CAN, USING THE PENCIL.

NOW ERASE IT. EASY, RIGHT?

STARE INTO THE ABYSS FOR A FEW
MINUTES AND SEE WHAT STARES BACK

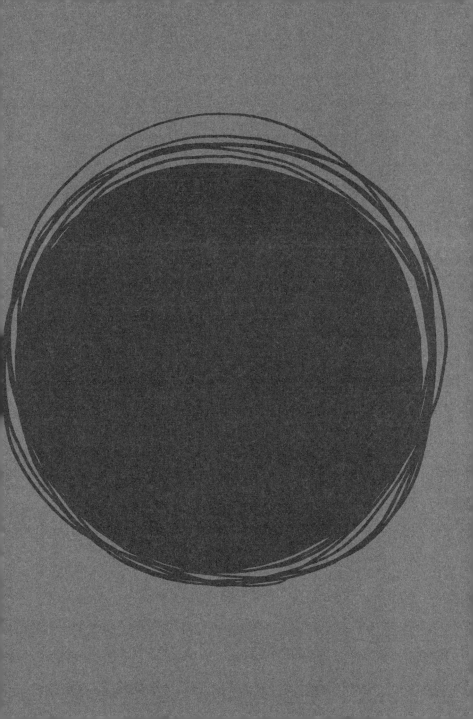

WHAT WOULD YOU SAVE IN A FIRE?

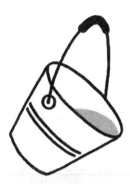

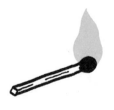

WHAT WOULD YOU BURN TO THE GROUND?

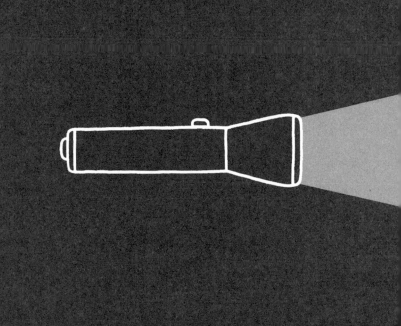

WRITE DOWN THE THOUGHTS YOU WANT
TO KEEP HIDING IN THE DARKNESS...

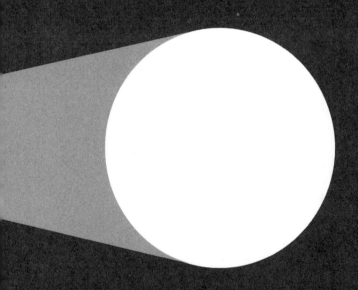

THEN SCRIBBLE OUT THE LIGHT

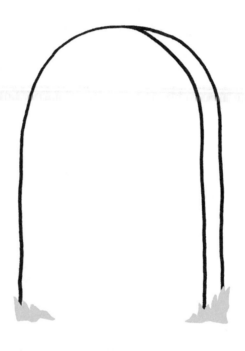

WHAT WILL YOU BE REMEMBERED FOR?

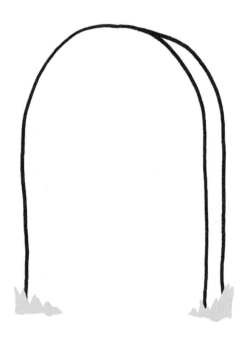

WHAT WOULD YOU LIKE TO BE REMEMBERED FOR?

ARE

LIVIN

EXIS

YOU

G OR

TING?

It can
be annoying when
life's big questions start to
circle around your mind as you should
be falling asleep: What am I doing with my
life? Where am I going? Is ice cream really that
bad for me? But that's your brain reminding you
that even though it's easy to forget about yourself,
it's important that you don't. The best time for you to
reconnect with your truest self is under the cover of
darkness. While the rest of the world is sleeping you
can be the most honest, ambitious, and free version
of yourself without worry or guilt. When the sun
rises you will again be the version of you that
people know and love, but armed with a
fresh energy and perspective about what
you want, where you are going,
and who you are.

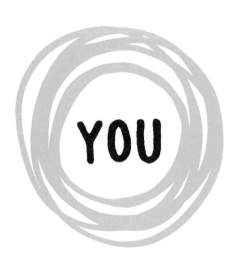

YOU

WHO ARE THE MOST IMPORTANT PEOPLE IN YOUR LIFE, AND WHAT DO THEY DO FOR YOU?

WHAT DO YOU DO FOR THEM?

PUT THE SYMBOLS BELOW ONTO THIS MAP

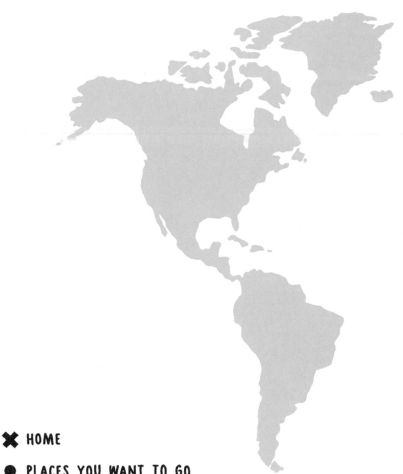

✖ HOME

● PLACES YOU WANT TO GO

★ YOUR FAVORITE PLACES

♥ THE PERSON YOU LOVE MOST

▲ THE FARTHEST YOU'VE BEEN FROM HOME

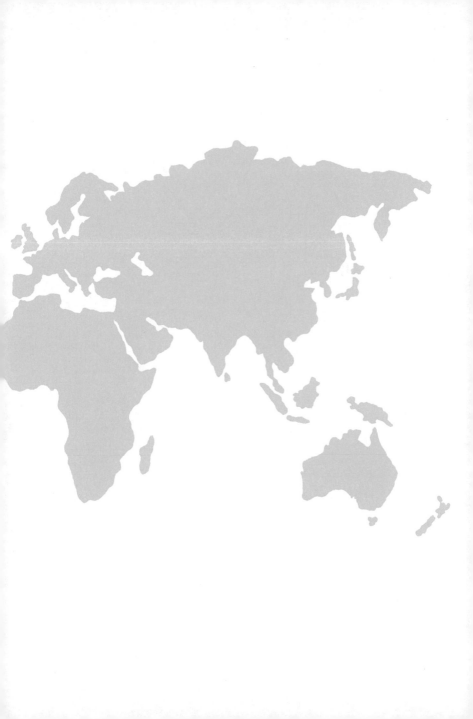

IMAGINE YOU'RE A BUILDING...
WHERE ARE YOU?

WHAT DO YOU LOOK LIKE?

WHAT IS YOUR PURPOSE?

RE THERE PEOPLE INSIDE YOU? WHAT DO THEY DO?

HAT CAN YOU SEE?

OW DO YOU FEEL?

THIS LIGHT IS SHINING ON YOUR
BEST QUALITY. WHAT IS IT?

WHAT IS YOUR PURPOSE?

WHAT IS THE POINT?

WHAT JOB DID YOU WANT AS A CHILD?

WOULD THE CURRENT VERSION
OF YOU BE HAPPY DOING THIS?

WHAT JOB DO YOU HAVE NOW?

WOULD THE CHILDHOOD VERSION OF YOU BE HAPPY DOING THIS?

WHAT WERE YOUR FAVORITE THINGS TO DO AS A CHILD?

WHICH OF THESE THINGS DO YOU NO LONGER DO?

WHEN DID YOU STOP DOING THEM?

WHY DID YOU STOP DOING THEM?

WHICH OF THEM DO YOU THINK YOU'D STILL ENJOY?

WHAT'S STOPPING YOU FROM DOING THEM AGAIN?

WRITE A LETTER TO YOURSELF IN 30 YEARS' TIME

TURN THIS SILHOUETTE INTO A SELF-PORTRAIT

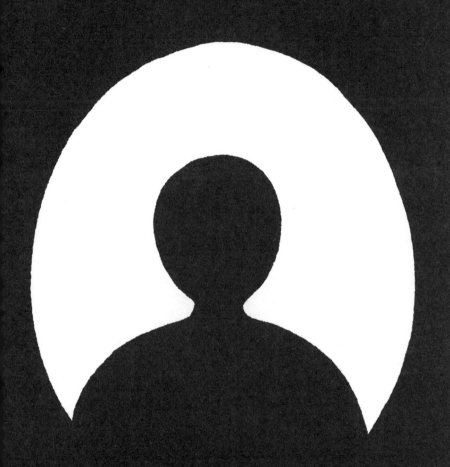

TURN THIS INTO SOMEONE YOU LOVE

WHAT THREE THINGS CHANGED YOUR LIFE THE MOST?

HOW DID THEY CHANGE YOUR LIFE?

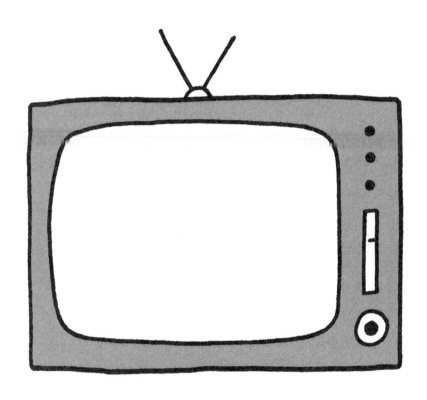

DESIGN THE TITLES FOR THE
TV SHOW ABOUT YOUR LIFE

WRITE A CAST LIST FOR THIS SHOW

ME ....

WHAT'S THE ONE THING THAT
ABSOLUTELY NO ONE KNOWS ABOUT YOU?

WHY HAVEN'T YOU TOLD ANYONE ABOUT IT?

WRITE IT ANONYMOUSLY ON A PIECE OF PAPER AND
HIDE IT IN A PLACE WHERE SOMEONE WILL FIND IT

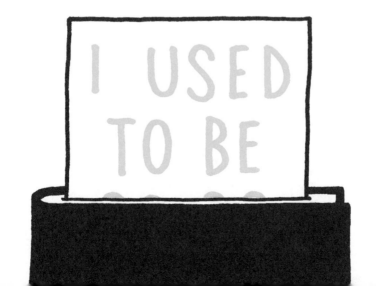

TURN THIS INTO A PIE CHART
OF HOW YOU SPENT YOUR DAY

IF YOU REPEATED THIS DAY FOR THE NEXT FIVE YEARS, WHERE WOULD YOU BE?

WHERE DO YOU WANT TO BE IN FIVE YEARS' TIME?

MAKE ANOTHER CHART OF HOW TO SPEND
YOUR DAYS SO YOU CAN ACHIEVE THIS GOAL

IF YOU COULD ASK EVERYONE IN THE WORLD ONE QUESTION, WHAT WOULD IT BE?

START BY ASKING YOUR FRIENDS AND FAMILY, ALL OF YOUR EMAIL CONTACTS, YOUR TWITTER FOLLOWERS, AND ANYONE ELSE YOU MEET.

ANSWER THE TEN IMPORTANT QUESTIONS YOU WROTE EARLIER

1:

2:

3:

4:

5:

6:

7:

8:

9:

10:

WHAT
REALLY

DO YOU WANT?

THANKS AS ALWAYS TO THE PEOPLE I USUALLY THANK:

Who hopefully already know just how thankful I am, both to them and for them.

TO THESE PEOPLE & THINGS THAT I CAN'T THANK IN PERSON:

Dad, Ice Cream, Nick Cave, Berlin, NASA, The Ocean, Starlee Kine, The National, Cheeseburgers, Miranda July, Sadness, Dinosaurs, Fleabag, Bonnie "Prince" Billy, London, The Goonies, Louis CK, South Africa, Erlend Loe, The "Beautiful Losers," Francis Mallmann, The Color Orange, You.

AND SPECIAL THANKS TO JAYNE.

FOLLOW @LEECRUTCHLEY OR VISIT LEECRUTCHLEY.COM

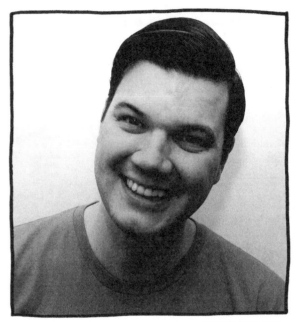

PHOTO BY JAYNE YONG

Lee Crutchley is an artist and author from England who is currently based in Berlin. His previous books have been translated into nineteen languages, and he is embarrassed to admit that he can only speak one. *Obwohl er sein Bestes gibt, um Deutsch zu lernen.*

ALSO BY LEE CRUTCHLEY

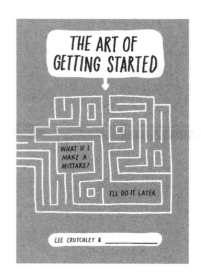

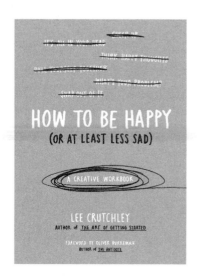

The Art of Getting Started

Whether it's perfectionism, procrastination, or plain old fear that's holding you back, get ready to get inspired!

How to Be Happy (Or at Least Less Sad)

Discover, explore, and remember all of those things that can make you feel happy...or at least less sad.

Find out more at **books.LeeCrutchley.com**